RENAL DIET

COOKBOOK

FISH SEAFOOD AND POULTRY

EDITION

A SCIENCE-BASED FOOD GUIDE WITH LOW SODIUM, LOW
POTASSIUM & LOW PHOSPHORUS TASTY RECIPES

ERICA WHITMAN

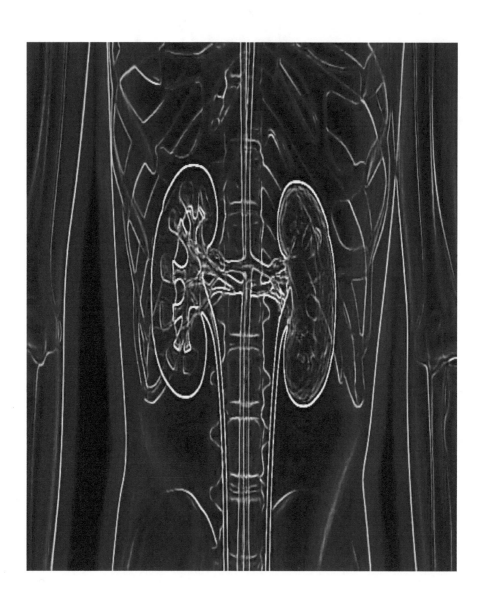

© **Copyright 2021 by Erica Whitman - All rights reserved.**

The following Book is reproduced below with the goal of providing information that is as accurate and reliable as possible. Regardless, purchasing this Book can be seen as consent to the fact that both the publisher and the author of this book are in no way experts on the topics discussed within and that any recommendations or suggestions that are made herein are for entertainment purposes only. Professionals should be consulted as needed prior to undertaking any of the action endorsed herein.

This declaration is deemed fair and valid by both the American Bar Association and the Committee of Publishers Association and is legally binding throughout the United States.

Furthermore, the transmission, duplication, or reproduction of any of the following work including specific information will be considered an illegal act irrespective of if it is done electronically or in print. This extends to creating a secondary or tertiary copy of the work or a recorded copy and is only allowed with the express written consent from the Publisher. All additional right reserved.

The information in the following pages is broadly considered a truthful and accurate account of facts and as such, any inattention, use, or misuse of the information in question by the reader will render any resulting actions solely under their purview. There are no scenarios in which the publisher or the original author of this work can be in any fashion deemed liable for any hardship or damages that may befall them after undertaking information described herein.

Additionally, the information in the following pages is intended only for informational purposes and should thus be thought of as universal. As befitting its nature, it is presented without assurance regarding its prolonged validity or interim quality. Trademarks that are mentioned are done without written consent and can in no way be considered an endorsement from the trademark holder.

Introduction

When we get sick, we tend to search for medication or a prescribed remedy to help our bodies fight whatever is wrong. When you're faced with something as subtle as a cold or flu, it's relatively easy to be aware of what you should eat to feel better. Usually, you are recommended to drink many fluids, primarily water, dose up on vitamins, ginger, honey, and herbs. Apart from medication prescribed by your doctor or pharmacist, what you eat and drink are two of the most important variables that can help you fight what is commonly known as influenza or any other infections relative to it.

With healing the body, humans tend to reach for medication before looking at their diets. For someone with a serious condition, like kidney disease or any other type of organ-derivative disease, eating the right type of food in proportion with the prescribed medication or treatment is significant.

Kidney disease is a severe disease that affects a person's entire life. It needs to be addressed and managed every day to ensure that the patient's condition doesn't deteriorate. Someone with kidney disease needs to address their diet to feel better and ensure their medication is also working effectively.

That's where the renal diet comes in. Renal diet is known for its effectiveness in conjunction with managing kidney disease and supporting a compulsory treatment for some patients, known as dialysis.

Kidney disease can reach a severe point. It can be a grueling and energy depriving experience. However, if you change your diet and adjust your eating habits to become healthier, you will have a much better experience managing your disease.

The Renal Diet Cookbook will provide you with everything you need to know to fight the effects of kidney disease and help you manage your well-being appropriately on your road to recovery.

Sodium, Potassium, And Phosphorus: Roles in Our Body

Sodium A mineral that helps regulate your body's water content and blood pressure is sodium. Healthy kidneys can remove sodium from the body as needed, but when your kidneys do not work well, sodium can build up and can cause high blood pressure, fluid-weight gain, and thirst. High blood pressure increases the chance of your kidney disease getting worse. If you are in the early stages of chronic kidney disease (stages 1 to 4), you will need to make some dietary modifications if you have high blood pressure or if you are retaining fluid. If you are experiencing stage five chronic kidney disease and require dialysis, you will need to follow a low-sodium diet and not consume more than 1,500 milligrams of sodium each day, which is equivalent to a little less than 1 teaspoon of salt. (It is important to note 1 teaspoon of salt each day is the total amount of sodium you are allowed, which includes all foods plus added salt.) Follow a sodium-restricted diet carefully to keep your blood pressure under control. Controlling your blood pressure may also prevent your risk of developing heart disease and decrease the chances of your kidney disease getting worse.

Potassium

You need potassium in your body to keep your heart strong and healthy. It is also needed to keep the water balance between your cells and body fluids in check. Healthy kidneys remove excess potassium through urination. The reason why kidneys are not functioning properly is they cannot remove the potassium, so it builds up in the blood.

While some people with kidney disease need more potassium, others need less. Depending on how well your kidneys are functioning, your potassium need may vary.

All foods contain some potassium, but some foods contain large amounts of potassium. On the following pages is a table that lists low-potassium, medium-potassium, and high-potassium foods. If you have chronic kidney disease, the amount of potassium you eat is not usually restricted unless your blood potassium level is high. Please talk with your physician about having your blood potassium level checked. And if you are receiving dialysis, your potassium intake should be kept between 2,000 and 3,000 milligrams per day.

Phosphorus

Phosphorus is a naturally occurring mineral. Phosphates are salt compounds containing phosphorus and other minerals, and these are found in our bones. Along with calcium, phosphorus helps build strong and healthy bones. Healthy kidneys are able to remove extra phosphorus in the blood. Virtually all foods have phosphorus or phosphate additives, so it is difficult to eliminate it from your diet completely.

If you excess phosphorus in your blood, calcium is pulled from your bones, resulting in weak bones. When the kidneys are failing, phosphorus builds up in the blood and may cause problems such as severe itching, muscle aches and pain, bone disease, and hardening of the blood vessels, including those leading to the heart, as well as deposits on the skin and in the joints.

FISH AND SEAFOOD RECIPES

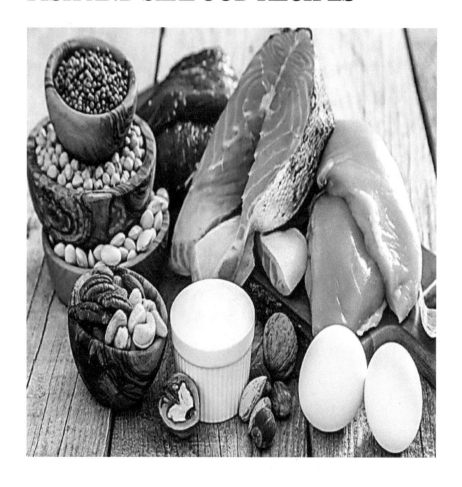

Seafood Casserole

Preparation Time: 20 minutes

Cooking Time: 45 minutes

Servings: 6

Ingredients:

Eggplant – 2 cups, peeled and diced into 1-inch pieces

Butter, for greasing the baking dish

Olive oil – 1 tbsp.

Sweet onion – ½, chopped

Minced garlic - 1 tsp.

Celery stalk – 1, chopped

Red bell pepper – ½, boiled and chopped

Freshly squeezed lemon juice – 3 Tbsps.

Hot sauce – 1 tsp.

Creole seasoning mix – ¼ tsp.

White rice – ½ cup, uncooked

Egg – 1 large

Cooked shrimp – 4 ounces

Queen crab meat – 6 ounces

Directions:

Preheat the oven to 350F.

Boil the eggplant in a saucepan for 5 minutes. Drain and set aside.

Grease a 9-by-13-inch baking dish with butter and set aside.

Heat the olive oil in a large skillet over medium heat.

Sauté the garlic, onion, celery, and bell pepper for 4 minutes or until tender.

Add the sautéed vegetables to the eggplant, along with the lemon juice, hot sauce, seasoning, rice, and egg.

Stir to combine.

Fold in the shrimp and crab meat.

Spoon the casserole mixture into the casserole dish, patting down the top.

Bake for 25 to 30 minutes or until casserole is heated through and rice is tender.

Serve warm.

Nutrition:

Calories: 118

Fat: 4g

Carb: 9g

Phosphorus: 102mg

Potassium: 199mg

Sodium: 235mg

Protein: 12g

Baked Trout

Preparation Time: 5 minutes

Cooking Time: 10 minutes

Servings: 8

Ingredients:

2-pound trout fillet

1 tablespoon oil

1 teaspoon salt-free lemon pepper

1/2 teaspoon paprika

Directions:

Preheat your oven to 350 degrees F.

Coat fillet with oil.

Place fish on a baking pan.

Season with lemon pepper and paprika.

Bake for 10 minutes.

Nutrition:

Calories 161

Protein 21 g

Carbohydrates 0 g

Fat 8 g

Cholesterol 58 mg

Sodium 109 mg

Potassium 385 mg

Phosphorus 227 mg

Calcium 75 mg

Fiber 0.1 g

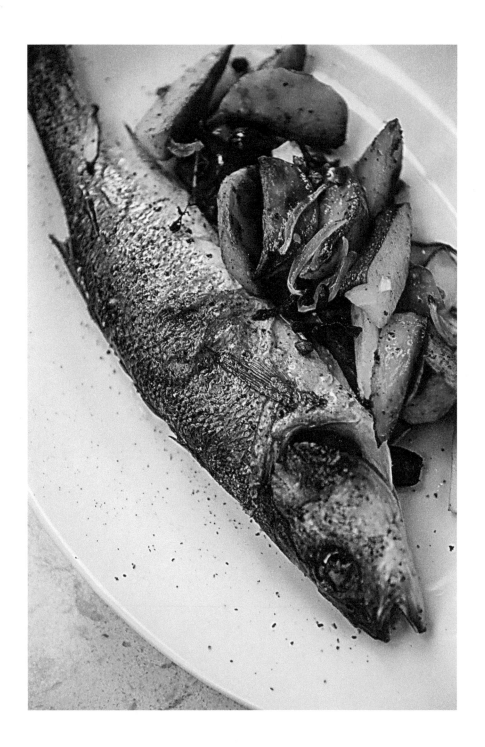

Shrimp in Garlic Sauce

Preparation Time: 10 minutes

Cooking Time: 6 minutes

Servings: 4

Ingredients:

3 tablespoons butter (unsalted)

1/4 cup onion, minced

3 cloves garlic, minced

1-pound shrimp, shelled and deveined

1/2 cup half and half creamer

1/4 cup white wine

2 tablespoons fresh basil

Black pepper to taste

Directions:

Add butter to a pan over medium low heat.

Let it melt.

Add the onion and garlic.

Cook for it 1-2 minutes.

Add the shrimp and cook for 2 minutes.

Transfer shrimp on a serving platter and set aside.

Add the rest of the ingredients.

Simmer for 3 minutes.

Pour sauce over the shrimp and serve.

Nutrition:

Calories 482

Protein 33 g

Carbohydrates 46 g

Fat 11 g

Cholesterol 230 mg

Sodium 213 mg

Potassium 514 mg

Phosphorus 398 mg

Calcium 133 mg

Fiber 2.0 g

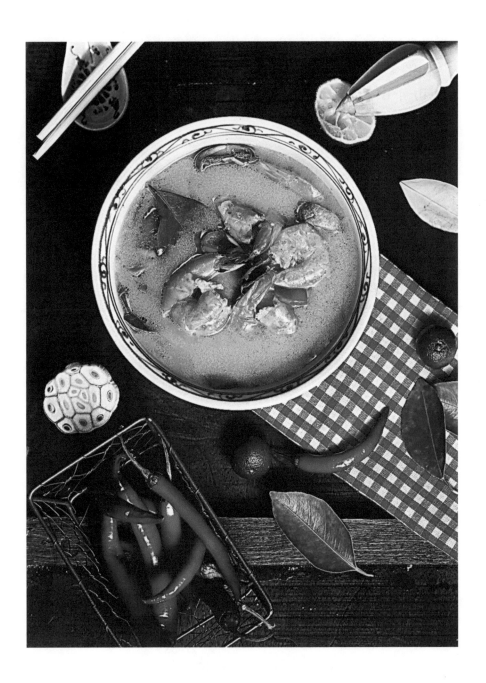

Fish Taco

Preparation Time: 40 minutes

Cooking Time: 10 minutes

Servings: 6

Ingredients:

1 tablespoon lime juice

1 tablespoon olive oil

1 clove garlic, minced

1-pound cod fillets

1/2 teaspoon ground cumin

1/4 teaspoon black pepper

1/2 teaspoon chili powder

1/4 cup sour cream

1/2 cup mayonnaise

2 tablespoons nondairy milk

1 cup cabbage, shredded

1/2 cup onion, chopped

1/2 bunch cilantro, chopped

12 corn tortillas

Directions:

Drizzle lemon juice over the fish fillet.

And then coat it with olive oil and then season with garlic, cumin, pepper and chili powder.

Let it sit for 30 minutes.

Broil fish for 10 minutes, flipping halfway through.

Flake the fish using a fork.

In a bowl, mix sour cream, milk and mayo.

Assemble tacos by filling each tortilla with mayo mixture, cabbage, onion, cilantro and fish flakes.

Nutrition:

Calories 366

Protein 18 g

Carbohydrates 31 g

Fat 19 g

Cholesterol 40 mg

Sodium 194 mg

Potassium 507 mg

Phosphorus 327 mg

Calcium 138 mg

Fiber 4.3 g

Salmon with Maple Glaze

Preparation Time: 15 minutes

Cooking Time: 2 hours

Servings: 4

Ingredients:

1-pound salmon fillets

1 tablespoon green onion, chopped

1 tablespoon low sodium soy sauce

2 garlic cloves, pressed

2 tablespoon fresh cilantro

3 tablespoon lemon juice (or juice of 1 lemon)

3 tablespoon maple syrup

Directions:

Combine all ingredients except for salmon.

Put salmon on platter and then pour marinade over fillets. Let it marinate 2 hours or more.

Preheat broiler.

Remove salmon from marinade.

Place salmon on bottom rack and broil for 10 minutes. Do not turn over.

Serve hot/cold with a wedge of lemon.

Nutrition:

Calories:220;

Carbs: 12g;

Protein: 24g;

Fats: 8g;

Phosphorus: 374mg;

Potassium: 440mg;

Sodium: 621mg

Baked Cod Crusted with Herbs

Preparation Time: 15 minutes

Cooking Time: 10 minutes

Servings: 4

Ingredients:

¼ cup honey

½ cup panko

½ teaspoon pepper

1 tablespoon extra-virgin olive oil

1 tablespoon lemon juice

1 teaspoon dried basil

1 teaspoon dried parsley

1 teaspoon rosemary

4 pieces of 4-ounce cod fillets

Directions:

With olive oil, grease a 9 x 13-inch baking pan and preheat oven to 375oF.

In a zip top bag mix panko, rosemary, pepper, parsley and basil.

Evenly spread cod fillets in prepped dish and drizzle with lemon juice.

Then brush the fillets with honey on all sides. Discard remaining honey if any.

Then evenly divide the panko mixture on top of cod fillets.

Pop in the oven and bake for ten minutes or until fish is cooked.

Serve and enjoy.

Nutrition:

Calories:113;

Carbs: 21g;

Protein: 5g;

Fats: 2g;

Phosphorus: 89mg;

Potassium: 115mg;

Sodium: 139mg

Dill Relish on White Sea Bass

Preparation Time: 15 minutes

Cooking Time: 60 minutes

Servings: 4

Ingredients:

1 lemon, quartered

4 pieces of 4-ounce white sea bass fillets

1 teaspoon lemon juice

1 teaspoon Dijon mustard

1 ½ teaspoons. chopped fresh dill

1 teaspoon pickled baby capers, drained

1 ½ tablespoons. chopped white onion

Directions:

Preheat oven to 3750F.

Mix lemon juice, mustard, dill, capers and onions in a small bowl.

Prepare four aluminum foil squares and place 1 fillet per foil.

Squeeze a lemon wedge per fish.

Evenly divide into 4 the dill spread and drizzle over fillet.

Close the foil over the fish securely and pop in the oven.

Bake for 9 to 12 minutes or until fish is cooked through.

Remove from foil and transfer to a serving platter, serve and enjoy.

Nutrition:

Calories:71;

Carbs: 11g;

Protein: 7g;

Fats: 1g;

Phosphorus: 91mg;

Potassium: 237mg;

Sodium: 94mg

Tilapia with Lemon Garlic Sauce

Preparation Time: 15 minutes

Cooking Time: 30 minutes

Servings: 4

Ingredients:

Pepper

1 teaspoon dried parsley flakes

1 clove garlic (finely chopped)

1 tablespoon butter (melted)

3 tablespoons. fresh lemon juice

4 tilapia fillets

Directions:

First, spray baking dish with non-stick cooking spray then preheat oven at 375 degrees Fahrenheit (190oC).

In cool water, rinse tilapia fillets and using paper towels pat dry the fillets.

Place tilapia fillets in the baking dish then pour butter and lemon juice and top off with pepper, parsley and garlic.

Bake tilapia in the preheated oven for 30 minutes and wait until fish is white.

Enjoy!

Nutrition:

Calories:168;

Carbs: 4g;

Protein: 24g;

Fats: 5g;

Phosphorus: 207mg;

Potassium: 431mg;

Sodium: 85mg

Lemon Butter Salmon

Preparation Time: 15 minutes

Cooking Time: 15 minutes

Servings: 6

Ingredients:

1 tablespoon butter

2 tablespoons olive oil

1 tablespoon Dijon mustard

1 tablespoons lemon juice

2 cloves garlic, crushed

1 teaspoon dried dill

1 teaspoon dried basil leaves

1 tablespoon capers

24-ounce salmon filet

Directions:

Put all of the ingredients except the salmon in a saucepan over medium heat.

Bring to a boil and then simmer for 5 minutes.

Preheat your grill.

Create a packet using foil.

Place the sauce and salmon inside.

Seal the packet.

Grill for 12 minutes.

Nutrition:

Calories 292

Protein 22 g

Carbohydrates 2 g

Fat 22 g

Cholesterol 68 mg

Sodium 190 mg

Potassium 439 mg

Phosphorus 280 mg

Calcium 21 mg

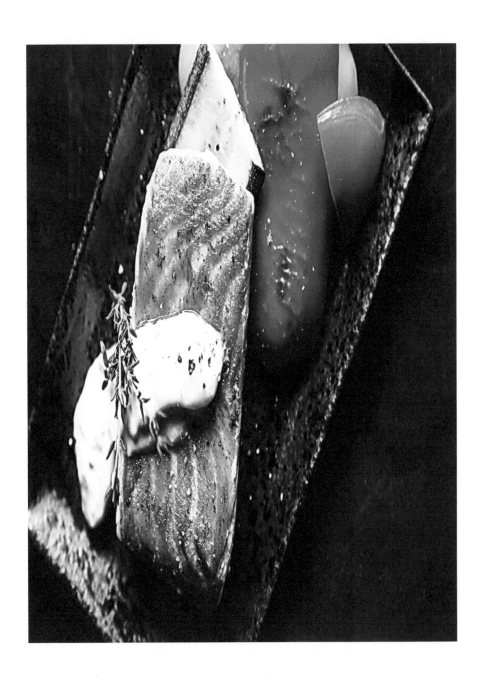

Crab Cake

Preparation Time: 15 minutes

Cooking Time: 9 minutes

Servings: 6

Ingredients:

1/4 cup onion, chopped

1/4 cup bell pepper, chopped

1 egg, beaten

6 low-sodium crackers, crushed

1/4 cup low-fat mayonnaise

1-pound crab meat

1 tablespoon dry mustard

Pepper to taste

2 tablespoons lemon juice

1 tablespoon fresh parsley

1 tablespoon garlic powder

3 tablespoons olive oil

Directions:

Mix all the ingredients except the oil.

Form 6 patties from the mixture.

Pour the oil into a pan in a medium heat.

Cook the crab cakes for 5 minutes.

Flip and cook for another 4 minutes.

Nutrition:

Calories 189

Protein 13 g

Carbohydrates 5 g

Fat 14 g

Cholesterol 111 mg

Sodium 342 mg

Potassium 317 mg

Phosphorus 185 mg

Calcium 52 mg

Fiber 0.5 g

Baked Fish in Cream Sauce

Preparation Time: 10 minutes

Cooking Time: 40 minutes

Servings: 4

Ingredients:

1-pound haddock

1/2 cup all-purpose flour

2 tablespoons butter (unsalted)

1/4 teaspoon pepper

2 cups fat-free nondairy creamer

1/4 cup water

Directions:

Preheat your oven to 350 degrees F.

Spray baking pan with oil.

Sprinkle with a little flour.

Arrange fish on the pan

Season with pepper.

Sprinkle remaining flour on the fish.

Spread creamer on both sides of the fish.

Bake for 40 minutes or until golden.

Spread cream sauce on top of the fish before serving.

Nutrition:

Calories 383

Protein 24 g

Carbohydrates 46 g

Fat 11 g

Cholesterol 79 mg

Sodium 253 mg

Potassium 400 mg

Phosphorus 266 mg

Calcium 46 mg

Fiber 0.4 g

Shrimp & Broccoli

Preparation Time: 10 minutes

Cooking Time: 5 minutes

Servings: 4

Ingredients:

1 tablespoon olive oil

1 clove garlic, minced

1-pound shrimp

1/4 cup red bell pepper

1 cup broccoli florets, steamed

10-ounce cream cheese

1/2 teaspoon garlic powder

1/4 cup lemon juice

3/4 teaspoon ground peppercorns

1/4 cup half and half creamer

Directions:

Pour the oil and cook garlic for 30 seconds.

Add shrimp and cook for 2 minutes.

Add the rest of the ingredients.

Mix well.

Cook for 2 minutes.

Nutrition:

Calories 469

Protein 28 g

Carbohydrates 28 g

Fat 28 g

Cholesterol 213 mg

Sodium 374 mg

Potassium 469 mg

Phosphorus 335 mg

Calcium 157 mg

Fiber 2.6 g

Fish with Mushrooms

Preparation Time: 5 minutes

Cooking Time: 16 minutes

Servings: 4

Ingredients:

1-pound cod fillet

2 tablespoons butter

¼ cup white onion, chopped

1 cup fresh mushrooms

1 teaspoon dried thyme

Directions:

Put the fish in a baking pan.

Preheat your oven to 450 degrees F.

Melt the butter and cook onion and mushroom for 1 minute.

Spread mushroom mixture on top of the fish.

Season with thyme.

Bake in the oven for 15 minutes.

Nutrition:

Calories 156

Protein 21 g

Carbohydrates 3 g

Fat 7 g

Cholesterol 49 mg

Sodium 110 mg

Potassium 561 mg

Phosphorus 225 mg

Calcium 30 mg

Fiber 0.5 g

Salmon with Spicy Honey

Preparation Time: 15 minutes

Cooking Time: 8 minutes

Servings: 2

Ingredients:

16-ounce salmon fillet

3 tablespoon honey

3/4 teaspoon lemon peel

3 bowls arugula salad

1/2 teaspoon black pepper

1/2 teaspoon garlic powder

2 teaspoon olive oil

1 teaspoon hot water

Directions:

Prepare a small bowl with some hot water and put in honey, grated lemon peel, ground pepper, and garlic powder.

Spread the mixture over salmon fillets.

Warm some olive oil at a medium heat and add spiced salmon fillet and cook for 4 minutes.

Turn the fillets on one side then on the other side.

Continue to cook for other 4 minutes at a reduced heat and try to check when the salmon fillets flake easily.

Put some arugula on each plate and add the salmon fillets on top, adding some aromatic herbs or some dill. Serve and enjoy!

Nutrition:

Calories: 320

Protein: 23 g

Sodium: 65 mg

Potassium: 450 mg

Phosphorus: 250 mg

Steamed Spicy Tilapia Fillet

Preparation Time: 10 minutes

Cooking Time: 25 minutes

Servings: 4

Ingredients:

4 fillets of tilapia

1 teaspoon hot pepper sauce

1 large sprig thyme

1 tablespoon Ketchup

1 tablespoon lime juice

1 cup hot water

1/2 cup onion, sliced

1/4 teaspoon black pepper

3/4 cup red and green peppers, sliced

Directions:

In a large shallow dish that fits your steamer, mix well hot pepper sauce, thyme, ketchup, lemon juice, and black pepper. Mix thoroughly.

Add tilapia fillets and spoon over sauce.

Mix in remaining ingredients except for water. Mix well in sauce.

Cover top of dish with foil.

Add the hot water in the steamer. Place dish on steamer rack.

Cover pot and steam fish and veggies for 20 minutes.

Let it stand for 5-6 minutes before serving.

Nutrition:

Calories:131;

Carbs: 5g;

Protein: 24g;

Fats: 3g;

Phosphorus: 212mg;

Potassium: 457mg;

Sodium: 102mg

Dijon Mustard and Lime Marinated Shrimp

Preparation Time: 20 minutes

Cooking Time: 80 minutes

Servings: 8

Ingredients:

1-pound uncooked shrimp, peeled and deveined

1 bay leaf

3 whole cloves

½ cup rice vinegar

1 cup water

½ teaspoon hot sauce

2 tablespoons. capers

2 tablespoons. Dijon mustard

½ cup fresh lime juice, plus lime zest as garnish

1 medium red onion, chopped

Directions:

Mix hot sauce, mustard, capers, lime juice and onion in a shallow baking dish and set aside.

Bring it to a boil in a large saucepan bay leaf, cloves, vinegar and water.

Once boiling, add shrimps and cook for a minute while stirring continuously.

Drain shrimps and pour shrimps into onion mixture.

For an hour, refrigerate while covered the shrimps.

Then serve shrimps cold and garnished with lime zest.

Nutrition:

Calories:123;

Carbs: 3g;

Protein: 12g;

Fats: 1g;

Phosphorus: 119mg;

Potassium: 87mg;

Sodium: 568mg

Spinach with Tuscan White Beans and Shrimps

Preparation Time: 5 minutes

Cooking Time: 15 minutes

Servings: 4

Ingredients:

1 ½ ounces crumbled reduce-fat feta cheese

5 cups baby spinach

15 ounces can no salt added cannellini beans (rinsed and drained)

½ cup low sodium, fat-free chicken broth

2 tablespoons. balsamic vinegar

2 teaspoons. chopped fresh sage

4 cloves garlic (minced)

1 medium onion (chopped)

1-pound large shrimp (peeled and deveined)

2 tablespoons. olive oil

Directions:

Heat 1 teaspoon oil. Heat it over medium-high.

Then for about 2 to 3 minutes, cook the shrimps using the heated skillet then place them on a plate. Heat on the same skillet the sage, garlic, and onions then cook for about 4 minutes. Add and stir in vinegar for 30 seconds.

For about 2 minutes, add chicken broth. Then, add spinach and beans and cook for an additional 2 to 3 minutes.

Remove skillet then add and stir in cooked shrimps topped with feta cheese.

Serve and divide into 4 bowls. Enjoy!

Nutrition:

Calories:343;

Carbs: 21g;

Protein: 22g;

Fats: 11g;

Phosphorus: 400mg;

Potassium: 599mg;

Sodium: 766mg

POULTRY RECIPES

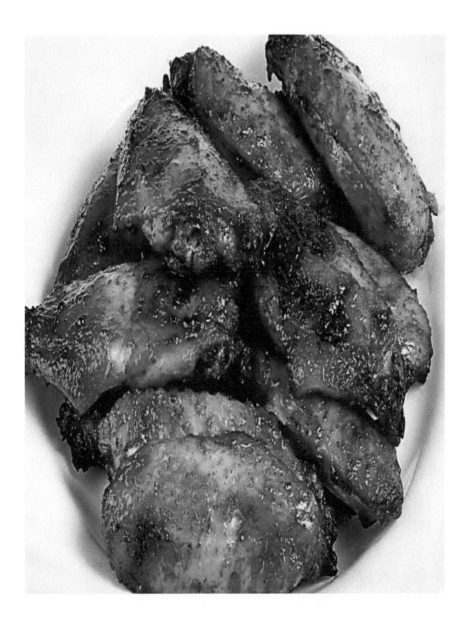

Chicken & Cauliflower Rice Casserole

Preparation Time: fifteen minutes

Cooking Time: an hour fifteen minutes

Servings: 8-10

Ingredients:

2 tablespoons coconut oil, divided

3-pound bone-in chicken thighs and drumsticks

Salt and freshly ground black pepper, to taste

3 carrots, peeled and sliced

1 onion, chopped finely

2 garlic cloves, chopped finely

2 tablespoons fresh cinnamon, chopped finely

2 teaspoons ground cumin

1 teaspoon ground coriander

12 teaspoon ground cinnamon

½ teaspoon ground turmeric

1 teaspoon paprika

¼ teaspoon red pepper cayenne

1 (28-ounce) can diced tomatoes with liquid

1 red bell pepper, seeded and cut into thin strips

½ cup fresh parsley leaves, minced

Salt, to taste

1 head cauliflower, grated to some rice like consistency

1 lemon, sliced thinly

Directions:

Preheat the oven to 375 degrees F.

In a large pan, melt 1 tablespoon of coconut oil high heat.

Add chicken pieces and cook for about 3-5 minutes per side or till golden brown.

Transfer the chicken in a plate.

In a similar pan, sauté the carrot, onion, garlic and ginger for about 4-5 minutes on medium heat.

Stir in spices and remaining coconut oil.

Add chicken, tomatoes, bell pepper, parsley and salt and simmer for approximately 3-5 minutes.

In the bottom of a 13x9-inch rectangular baking dish, spread the cauliflower rice evenly.

Place chicken mixture over cauliflower rice evenly and top with lemon slices.

With a foil paper, cover the baking dish and bake for approximately 35 minutes.

Uncover the baking dish and bake approximately 25 minutes.

Nutrition:

Calories: 412,

Fat: 12g,

Carbohydrates: 23g,

Fiber: 7g,

Protein: 34g

Phosphorus 297 mg

Potassium 811 mg

Sodium 711 mg

Chicken Meatloaf with Veggies

Preparation Time: 20 minutes

Cooking Time: 1-1¼ hours

Servings: 4

Ingredients:

For Meatloaf:

½ cup cooked chickpeas

2 egg whites

2½ teaspoons poultry seasoning

Salt and freshly ground black pepper, to taste

10-ounce lean ground chicken

1 cup red bell pepper, seeded and minced

1 cup celery stalk, minced

1/3 cup steel-cut oats

1 cup tomato puree, divided

2 tablespoons dried onion flakes, crushed

1 tablespoon prepared mustard

For Veggies:

2-pounds summer squash, sliced

16-ounce frozen Brussels sprouts

2 tablespoons extra-virgin extra virgin olive oil

Salt and freshly ground black pepper, to taste

Directions:

Preheat the oven to 350 degrees F. Grease a 9x5-inch loaf pan.

In a mixer, add chickpeas, egg whites, poultry seasoning, salt and black pepper and pulse till smooth.

Transfer a combination in a large bowl.

Add chicken, veggies oats, ½ cup of tomato puree and onion flakes and mix till well combined.

Transfer the amalgamation into prepared loaf pan evenly.

With both hands, press, down the amalgamation slightly.

In another bowl mix together mustard and remaining tomato puree.

Place the mustard mixture over loaf pan evenly.

Bake approximately 1-1¼ hours or till desired doneness.

Meanwhile in a big pan of water, arrange a steamer basket.

Bring to a boil and set summer time squash I steamer basket.

Cover and steam approximately 10-12 minutes.

Drain well and aside.

Now, prepare the Brussels sprouts according to package's directions.

In a big bowl, add veggies, oil, salt and black pepper and toss to coat well.

Serve the meatloaf with veggies.

Nutrition:

Calories: 420,

Fat: 9g,

Carbohydrates: 21g,

Fiber: 14g,

Protein: 36g

Phosphorus 431 mg

Potassium 472 mg

Sodium 249 mg

Basil Chicken

Preparation Time: 15 minutes

Cooking Time: 25 minutes

Servings: 4

Ingredients:

4 chicken breast fillets

1/4 cup butter, melted

1/4 teaspoon garlic powder

1/4 cup fresh basil

1/4 teaspoon herb seasoning blend

1 tablespoon Parmesan cheese, grated

Directions:

Preheat your oven to 325 degrees F.

Put the chicken breast fillet in a baking pan.

Combine butter, garlic powder, basil, herb seasoning and cheese.

Spread mixture over the chicken fillets, coating both sides.

Bake for 25 minutes.

Nutrition:

Calories 252

Protein 27 g

Carbohydrates 0 g

Fat 16 g

Cholesterol 74 mg

Sodium 231 mg

Potassium 246 mg

Phosphorus 210 mg

Calcium 31 mg

Fiber 0.1 g

Turkey with Curry Glaze

Preparation Time: 10 minutes

Cooking Time: 30 minutes

Serving: 8

Ingredients:

3 lb. turkey breast fillet

1/4 cup butter, melted

1/4 cup honey

1 tablespoon mustard

2 teaspoons curry powder

1 teaspoon garlic powder

Directions:

Add the turkey breast fillet on a roasting pan.

Bake at 350 degrees F in the oven for 1 hour.

While waiting, combine the rest of the ingredients in a bowl.

In the last 30 minutes of baking, brush the turkey breast with the mixture.

Let turkey sit for 15 minutes before slicing and serving.

Nutrition:

Calories 275

Protein 26 g

Carbohydrates 9 g

Fat 13 g

Cholesterol 82 mg

Sodium 122 mg

Potassium 277 mg

Phosphorus 193 mg

Calcium 24 mg

Fiber 0.2 g

Rosemary Chicken

Preparation Time: 20 minutes

Cooking Time: 45 minutes

Servings: 4

Ingredients:

1/2 onion, sliced into wedges

8 cloves garlic, crushed

1/2 bell pepper, sliced

1 carrots, sliced into rounds

2 zucchini, sliced into rounds

1 tablespoon olive oil

4 chicken breasts

1/4 teaspoon ground pepper

1 tablespoon dried rosemary

Directions:

Preheat your oven to 375 degrees F.

Toss the onion, garlic, bell pepper, carrot and zucchini in a roasting pan.

Drizzle with oil.

Roast in the oven for 10 minutes.

While waiting, season chicken with pepper and rosemary.

Put the chicken on top of the vegetables.

Put them back in the oven.

Bake for 35 minutes.

Nutrition:

Calories 215

Protein 30 g

Carbohydrates 8 g

Fat 7 g

Cholesterol 73 mg

Sodium 107 mg

Potassium 580 mg

Phosphorus 250 mg

Calcium 65 mg

Fiber 3.0 g

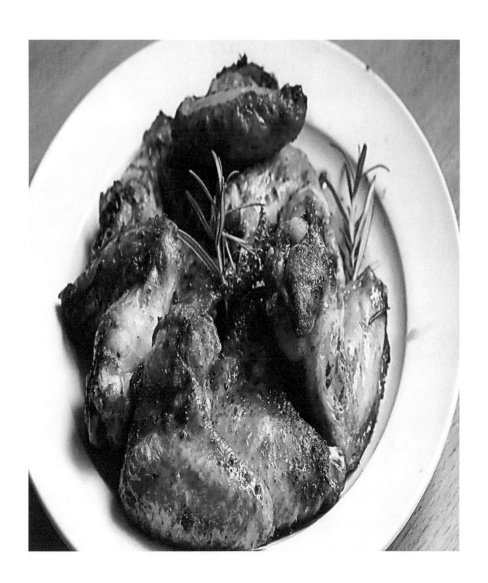

Apple and Chicken Curry

Preparation Time: 15 minutes

Cooking Time: 1 hour and 10 minutes

Servings: 8

Ingredients:

1 medium apple: peeled, cored, chopped

8 skinless chicken breast

1 small white onion, peeled and chopped

½ teaspoon minced garlic

3 tablespoons all-purpose white flour

½ tablespoon dried basil

¼ teaspoon ground black pepper

1 tablespoon curry powder

3 tablespoons unsalted butter

1 cup chicken broth, low-sodium

1 cup rice milk, unenriched

Directions:

Switch on the oven, then set it to 350°F and let it preheat.

Take a 9-by-13 inch baking dish, grease it with oil, place chicken in it in a single layer. Sprinkle with black pepper and set aside until required.

Take a medium-sized saucepan, place it over medium heat, add butter and when it melts, add onion and apple and cook for 5 minutes, or until tender.

Season with basil and curry powder, cook for 1 minute until saute, and then stir in flour, continue cooking for 1 minute.

Pour in milk and broth, stir until combined, remove the pan from heat, pour this sauce over chicken, and then bake for 60 minutes until thoroughly cooked.

Serve straight away.

Nutrition:

Calories – 232

Cholesterol – 85 ml

Fat – 8 g

Net Carbs – 9.8 g

Protein – 29 g

Sodium – 118 mg

Carbohydrates – 11 g

Potassium – 323 mg

Fiber – 1.2 g

Phosphorus – 225 mg

Chicken with Garlic Sauce

Preparation Time: 10 minutes

Cooking Time: 30 minutes

Servings: 8

Ingredients:

8 skinless chicken breasts

1 medium head of garlic, peeled and sliced

½ teaspoon ground black pepper

1 tablespoon rosemary leaves, chopped

½ cup balsamic vinegar

2 tablespoons olive oil

½ cup white wine

2 cups chicken broth, low-sodium

Directions:

Take a 9-by-13 inches baking dish, add rosemary, wine, and vinegar, pour in the broth, stir until mixed, add chicken, toss it well and let it marinate for a minimum of 4 hours.

Then take a large saute pan, place it over medium-high heat, add oil and when hot, add sliced garlic and cook for 4 minutes, or until golden.

Transfer garlic to a plate, set aside until needed, switch to high heat, add marinated chicken in it, sprinkle with black pepper, and cook for 1 minute per side until golden.

Then switch to medium heat, pour marinade over the chicken, add garlic and simmer the chicken for 15 minutes until cooked, turning halfway.

When done, transfer chicken to a dish, switch to high heat, and bring the sauce to a boil, then switch heat to medium-high and simmer the liquid until thickened.

Drizzle liquid over chicken and then serve.

Nutrition:

Calories – 210

Cholesterol – 70 ml

Fat – 7 g

Net Carbs – 3.8 g

Protein – 28 g

Sodium – 85 mg

Carbohydrates – 4 g

Potassium – 277 mg

Fiber – 0.2 g

Phosphorus – 208 mg

Chicken Pot Pie

Preparation Time: 10 minutes

Cooking Time: 1 hour and 15 minutes

Servings: 8

Ingredients:

12-ounce farfalle pasta

1 ½ cup carrots, sliced

2 pounds skinless chicken breasts

1 cup celery, diced

2 cups potatoes, diced

1 cup white onion, diced

12 cups water

¼ teaspoon ground black pepper

½ teaspoon dried thyme

2 tablespoons parsley, chopped

Directions:

Take a large saucepan, place it over medium-high heat, add chicken, stir in all the seasoning, pour in water, bring it to a boil, then switch to medium-low heat and simmer for 45 minutes.

Meanwhile, take a large pot, place it over medium-high heat, place potatoes in it, pour in water to cover the potatoes, and bring it to a boil.

Then drain the water, cover potatoes with fresh water, bring it to a boil, and continue cooking for 10 minutes. When done, drain the potatoes and set aside until required.

When the chicken has cooked, remove the pan from heat, then remove chicken from it and set aside until required.

Remove fat from the broth by skimming it, then place the pan over medium-high heat, add carrot, onion, and celery, bring it to a boil, and then cook for 5 minutes.

Add potatoes and pasta, stir in parsley, and boil for 14 minutes, or until pasta is tender.

Cut the chicken into bite-sized pieces, add into the pan, stir and cook until thoroughly heated.

Serve straight away.

Nutrition:

Calories – 335

Cholesterol – 70 ml

Fat – 4 g

Net Carbs – 38.7 g

Protein – 32 g

Sodium – 118 mg

Carbohydrates – 42 g

Potassium – 521 mg

Fiber – 3.3 g

Phosphorus – 290 mg

Sweet & Sour Chicken

Preparation Time: 15 minutes

Cooking Time: 20 minutes

Servings: 5

Ingredients:

1/4 cup apple cider vinegar

1 cup low-sodium chicken broth

1/4 cup brown sugar

1/2 teaspoon garlic, chopped

2 teaspoons low-sodium soy sauce

8 oz. canned pineapple chunks

1 lb. chicken breast, cubed

1 onion, diced

1 green bell pepper, sliced

1 cup celery, sliced

3 tablespoons cornstarch

1/4 cup water

Directions:

Get the juice from the pineapple chunks.

Pour pineapple juice, vinegar, broth, sugar, garlic and soy sauce into a pan over low heat.

Add the chicken.

Cover the pan and simmer for 15 minutes.

Add the pineapple chunks and the vegetables.

Thicken the sauce using a mix of water and cornstarch.

Nutrition:

Calories 310

Protein 24 g

Carbohydrates 47 g

Fat 3 g

Cholesterol 57 mg

Sodium 270 mg

Potassium 420 mg

Phosphorus 211 mg

Calcium 43 mg

Fiber 1.6 g

Turkey Meatloaf

Preparation Time: 15 minutes

Cooking Time: 1 hour

Servings: 6

Ingredients:

1 lb. ground turkey

3 ounces turkey sausage

1/2 cup dry breadcrumbs

2 eggs, beaten

1 tablespoon Worcestershire sauce

1 teaspoon Italian seasoning

1/4 cup fresh parsley, chopped

1/2 teaspoon black pepper

Directions:

Preheat your oven to 350 degrees F.

Put all the ingredients in a bowl and mix.

Press mixture into a loaf pan.

Bake for 1 hour.

Nutrition:

Calories 197

Protein 20 g

Carbohydrates 9 g

Fat 9 g

Cholesterol 85 mg

Sodium 305 mg

Potassium 314 mg

Phosphorus 206 mg

Calcium 49 mg

Fiber 0.4 g

Chicken Marsala

Preparation Time: 15 minutes

Cooking Time: 15 minutes

Servings: 4

Ingredients:

4 chicken breast fillets

1/2 cup all-purpose flour

2 tablespoons olive oil

1/2 cup shallots, chopped

2 cups fresh mushrooms, sliced

5 tablespoons fresh parsley, chopped

1 tablespoon butter mixed with 1 tablespoon olive oil

1/4 cup dry Marsala wine

1/4 teaspoon garlic powder

1/8 teaspoon black pepper

Directions:

Coat both sides of chicken with flour.

Cook in hot oil in a pan over medium heat.

Cook until golden or for 5 minutes per side.

Put chicken on a platter and set aside.

Sauté mushrooms, parsley and shallots in olive oil butter blend for 3 minutes.

Add the rest of the ingredients.

Simmer for 2 minutes.

Pour sauce over chicken and serve with rice.

Nutrition:

Calories 425

Protein 32 g

Carbohydrates 40 g

Fat 15 g

Cholesterol 70 mg

Sodium 145 mg

Potassium 480 mg

Phosphorus 300 mg

Calcium 46 mg

Fiber 2.0 g

Zesty Chicken

Preparation Time: 40 minutes

Cooking Time: 10 minutes

Servings: 2

Ingredients:

2 tablespoons olive oil

2 tablespoons balsamic vinegar

1/4 cup green onion, chopped

1 teaspoon fresh oregano

1/2 teaspoon garlic powder

1/4 teaspoon black pepper

1/4 teaspoon paprika

8 ounces chicken breast fillets

Directions:

Mix olive oil and vinegar.

Add green onion, herbs and seasonings.

Mix well.

Marinate chicken in the mixture for 30 minutes.

Cover and put inside the refrigerator.

Fry the chicken for 5 minutes per side.

Nutrition:

Calories 280

Protein 27 g

Carbohydrates 4 g

Fat 16 g

Cholesterol 73 mg

Sodium 68 mg

Potassium 280 mg

Phosphorus 205 mg

Calcium 26 mg

Fiber 0.3 g

Roasted Spatchcock Chicken

Preparation Time: twenty or so minutes

Cooking Time: 50 minutes

Servings: 4-6

Ingredients:

1 (4-pound) whole chicken

1 (1-inch) piece fresh ginger, sliced

4 garlic cloves, chopped

1 small bunch fresh thyme

Pinch of cayenne

Salt and freshly ground black pepper, to taste

¼ cup fresh lemon juice

3 tablespoons extra virgin olive oil

Directions:

Arrange chicken, breast side down onto a large cutting board.

With a kitchen shear, begin with thigh and cut along 1 side of backbone and turn chicken around.

Now, cut along sleep issues and discard the backbone.

Change the inside and open it like a book.

Flatten the backbone firmly to flatten.

In a food processor, add all ingredients except chicken and pulse till smooth.

In a big baking dish, add the marinade mixture.

Add chicken and coat with marinade generously.

With a plastic wrap, cover the baking dish and refrigerate to marinate for overnight.

Preheat the oven to 450 degrees F. Arrange a rack in a very roasting pan.

Remove the chicken from refrigerator make onto rack over roasting pan, skin side down.

Roast for about 50 minutes, turning once in the middle way.

Nutrition:

Calories: 419,

Fat: 14g,

Carbohydrates: 28g,

Fiber: 4g,

Protein: 40g

Phosphorus 281 mg

Potassium 354 mg

Sodium 165 mg

Avocado-Orange Grilled Chicken

Preparation Time: 20 minutes

Cooking Time: 60 minutes

Servings: 4

Ingredients:

¼ cup fresh lime juice

¼ cup minced red onion

1 avocado

1 cup low fat yogurt

1 small red onion, sliced thinly

1 tablespoon honey

2 oranges, peeled and sectioned

2 tablespoons. chopped cilantro

4 pieces of 4-6ounce boneless, skinless chicken breasts

Pepper and salt to taste

Directions:

In a large bowl mix honey, cilantro, minced red onion and yogurt.

Submerge chicken into mixture and marinate for at least 30 minutes.

Grease grate and preheat grill to medium high fire.

Remove chicken from marinade and season with pepper and salt.

Grill for 6 minutes per side or until chicken is cooked and juices run clear.

Meanwhile, peel avocado and discard seed. Chop avocados and place in bowl. Quickly add lime juice and toss avocado to coat well with juice.

Add cilantro, thinly sliced onions and oranges into bowl of avocado, mix well.

Serve grilled chicken and avocado dressing on the side.

Nutrition:

Calories: 209;

Carbs: 26g;

Protein: 8g;

Fats: 10g;

Phosphorus: 157mg;

 Potassium: 548mg;

Sodium: 125mg

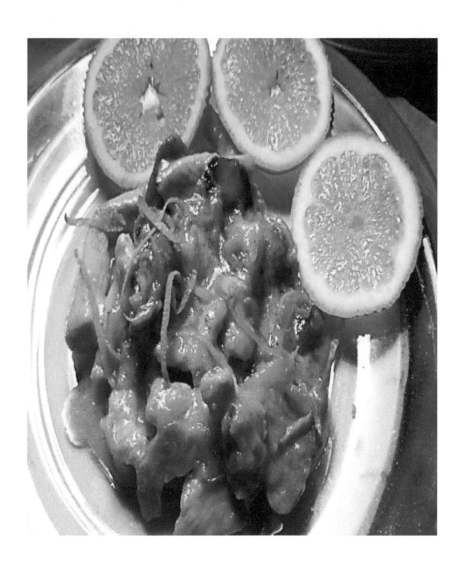

Ground Chicken & Peas Curry

Preparation Time: 15 minutes

Cooking Time: 6-10 minutes

Servings: 3-4

Ingredients:

For Marinade:

3 tablespoons essential olive oil

2 bay leaves

2 onions, grinded to some paste

½ tablespoon garlic paste

½ tablespoon ginger paste

2 tomatoes, chopped finely

1 tablespoon ground cumin

1 tablespoon ground coriander

1 teaspoon ground turmeric

1 teaspoon red chili powder

Salt, to taste

1-pound lean ground chicken

2 cups frozen peas

1½ cups water

1-2 teaspoons garam masala powder

Directions:

In a deep skillet, heat oil on medium heat.

Add bay leaves and sauté for approximately half a minute.

Add onion paste and sauté for approximately 3-4 minutes.

Add garlic and ginger paste and sauté for around 1-1½ minutes.

Add tomatoes and spices and cook, stirring occasionally for about 3-4 minutes.

Stir in chicken and cook for about 4-5 minutes.

Stir in peas and water and bring to a boil on high heat.

Reduce the heat to low and simmer approximately 5-8 minutes or till desired doneness.

Stir in garam masala and remove from heat.

Serve hot.

Nutrition:

Calories: 450,

Fat: 10g,

Carbohydrates: 19g,

Fiber: 6g,

Protein: 38g

Chicken Meatballs Curry

Preparation Time: 20 min

Cooking Time: 25 minutes

Servings: 3-4

Ingredients:

For Meatballs:

1-pound lean ground chicken

1 tablespoon onion paste

1 teaspoon fresh ginger paste

1 teaspoons garlic paste

1 green chili, chopped finely

1 tablespoon fresh cilantro leaves, chopped

1 teaspoon ground coriander

½ teaspoon cumin seeds

½ teaspoon red chili powder

½ teaspoon ground turmeric

Salt, to taste

For Curry:

3 tablespoons extra-virgin olive oil

½ teaspoon cumin seeds

1 (1-inch) cinnamon stick

3 whole cloves

3 whole green cardamoms

1 whole black cardamom

2 onions, chopped

1 teaspoon fresh ginger, minced

1 teaspoons garlic, minced

4 whole tomatoes, chopped finely

2 teaspoons ground coriander

1 teaspoon garam masala powder

½ teaspoon ground nutmeg

½ teaspoon red chili powder

½ teaspoon ground turmeric

Salt, to taste

1 cup water

Chopped fresh cilantro, for garnishing

Directions:

For meatballs in a substantial bowl, add all ingredients and mix till well combined.

Make small equal-sized meatballs from mixture.

In a big deep skillet, heat oil on medium heat.

Add meatballs and fry approximately 3-5 minutes or till browned from all sides.

Transfer the meatballs in a bowl.

In the same skillet, add cumin seeds, cinnamon stick, cloves, green cardamom and black cardamom and sauté approximately 1 minute.

Add onions and sauté for around 4-5 minutes.

Add ginger and garlic paste and sauté approximately 1 minute.

Add tomato and spices and cook, crushing with the back of spoon for approximately 2-3 minutes.

Add water and meatballs and provide to a boil.

Reduce heat to low.

Simmer for approximately 10 minutes.

Serve hot with all the garnishing of cilantro.

Nutrition:

Calories: 421,

Fat: 8g,

Carbohydrates: 18g,

Fiber: 5g,

Protein: 34g

Herbs and Lemony Roasted Chicken

Preparation Time: 15 minutes

Cooking Time: 1 ½ hours

Servings: 8

Ingredients:

½ teaspoon ground black pepper

½ teaspoon mustard powder

½ teaspoon salt

1 3-lb whole chicken

1 teaspoon garlic powder

2 lemons

2 tablespoons. olive oil

2 teaspoons. Italian seasoning

Directions:

In small bowl, mix well black pepper, garlic powder, mustard powder, and salt.

Rinse chicken well and slice off giblets.

In a greased 9 x 13 baking dish, place chicken and add 1 ½ teaspoons. of seasoning made earlier inside the chicken and rub the remaining seasoning around chicken.

In small bowl, mix olive oil and juice from 2 lemons. Drizzle over chicken.

Bake chicken in a preheated 3500F oven until juices run clear, around 1 ½ hours. Every once in a while, baste chicken with its juices.

Nutrition:

Calories: 190;

Carbs: 2g;

Protein: 35g;

Fats: 9g;

Phosphorus: 341mg;

Potassium: 439mg;

Sodium: 328mg

Creamy Mushroom and Broccoli Chicken

Preparation Time: 15 minutes

Cooking Time: 6 hours

Servings: 6

Ingredients:

1 10.5 ounce can of low-sodium cream of mushroom soup

1 21 ounce can of low-sodium cream of Chicken Soup

2 whole cooked chicken breasts, chopped or shredded

2 cup milk

1lb broccoli florets

¼ teaspoon garlic powder

Directions:

Place all ingredients to a 5 quart or larger slow cooker and mix well.

Cover and cook on LOW for 6 hours.

Serve with potatoes, pasta, or rice.

Nutrition:

Calories 155,

Fat 2g,

Carbs 19g,

Protein 12g,

Fiber 2g,

Potassium 755mg,

Sodium 35mg

Phosphorus 298 mg

Chicken Curry

Preparation Time: 10 minutes

Cooking Time: 4 minutes

Servings: 4

Ingredients:

1lb skinless chicken breasts

1 medium onion, thinly sliced

1 15 ounce can chickpeas, drained and rinsed well

2 medium sweet potatoes, peeled and diced

½ cup light coconut milk

½ cup chicken stock (see recipe)

1 15ounce can sodium-free tomato sauce

2 tablespoon curry powder

1 teaspoon low-sodium salt

½ cayenne powder

1 cup green peas

2 tablespoon lemon juice

Directions:

Place the chicken breasts, onion, chickpeas, and sweet potatoes into a 4 to 6-quart slow cooker.

Mix the coconut milk, chicken stock, tomato sauce, curry powder, salt, and cayenne together and pour into the slow cooker, stirring to coat well.

Cover and cook on Low for 8 hours or High for 4 hours.

Stir in the peas and lemon juice 5 minutes before serving.

Nutrition:

Calories 302,

Fat 5g,

Carbs 43g,

Protein 24g,

Fiber 9g,

Potassium 573mg,

Sodium 800mg

Phosphorus 416 mg

Ground Chicken with Basil

Preparation Time: 15 minutes

Cooking Time: 16 minutes

Servings: 8

Ingredients:

2 pounds lean ground chicken

3 tablespoons coconut oil, divided

1 zucchini, chopped

1 red bell pepper, seeded and chopped

½ of green bell pepper, seeded and chopped

4 garlic cloves, minced

1 (1-inch) piece fresh ginger, minced

1 (1-inch) piece fresh turmeric, minced

1 fresh red chile, sliced thinly

1 tablespoon organic honey

1 tablespoon coconut amino

1½ tablespoons fish sauce

½ cup fresh basil, chopped

Salt and freshly ground black pepper, to taste

1 tablespoon fresh lime juice

Directions:

Heat a large skillet on medium-high heat.

Add ground beef and cook for approximately 5 minutes or till browned completely.

Transfer the beef in a bowl.

In a similar pan, melt 1 tablespoon of coconut oil on medium-high heat.

Add zucchini and bell peppers and stir fry for around 3-4 minutes.

Transfer the vegetables inside bowl with chicken.

In exactly the same pan, melt remaining coconut oil on medium heat.

Add garlic, ginger, turmeric and red chile and sauté for approximately 1-2 minutes.

Add chicken mixture, honey and coconut amino and increase the heat to high.

Cook, stirring occasionally for approximately 4-5 minutes or till sauce is nearly reduced.

Stir in remaining ingredients and take off from heat.

Nutrition:

Calories: 407,

Fat: 7g,

Carbohydrates: 20g,

Fiber: 13g,

Protein: 36g

Phosphorus 210 mg

Potassium 645 mg

Sodium 336 mg

Asian Chicken Satay

Preparation Time: 15 minutes

Cooking Time: 10 minutes

Servings: 6

Ingredients:

Juice of 2 limes

Brown sugar – 2 tablespoons

Minced garlic – 1 tablespoon

Ground cumin – 2 teaspoons

Boneless, skinless chicken breast – 12, cut into strips

Directions:

In a bowl, stir together the cumin, garlic, brown sugar, and lime juice.

Add the chicken strips to the bowl and marinate in the refrigerator for 1 hour.

Heat the barbecue to medium-high.

Remove the chicken from the marinade and thread each strip onto wooden skewers that have been soaked in the water.

Grill the chicken for about 4 minutes per side or until the meat is cooked through but still juicy.

Nutrition:

Calories: 78

Carb: 4g

Phosphorus: 116mg

Potassium: 108mg

Sodium: 100mg

Protein: 12g

Zucchini and Turkey Burger with Jalapeno Peppers

Preparation Time: 15 minutes

Cooking Time: 10 minutes

Servings: 4

Ingredients:

Turkey meat (ground) – 1 pound

Zucchini (shredded) – 1 cup

Onion (minced) – ½ cup

Jalapeño pepper (seeded and minced) – 1

Egg – 1

Extra-spicy blend – 1 teaspoon

Fresh poblano peppers (seeded and sliced in half lengthwise)

Mustard – 1 teaspoon

Directions:

Start by taking a mixing bowl and adding in the turkey meat, zucchini, onion, jalapeño pepper, egg, and extra-spicy blend. Mix well to combine.

Divide the mixture into 4 equal portions. Form burger patties out of the same.

Prepare an electric griddle or an outdoor grill. Place the burger patties on the grill and cook until the top is blistered and tender. Place the sliced poblano peppers on the grill alongside the patties. Grilling the patties should take about 5 minutes on each side.

Once done, place the patties onto the buns and top them with grilled peppers.

Nutrition:

Protein – 25 g

Carbohydrates – 5 g

Fat – 10 g

Cholesterol – 125 mg

Sodium – 128 mg

Potassium – 475 mg

Phosphorus – 280 mg

Calcium – 43 mg

Fiber – 1.6 g

Chicken & Veggie Casserole

Preparation Time: 15 minutes

Cooking Time: half an hour

Servings: 4

Ingredients:

1/3 cup Dijon mustard

1/3 cup organic honey

1 teaspoon dried basil

¼ teaspoon ground turmeric

1 teaspoon dried basil, crushed

Salt and freshly ground black pepper, to taste

1¾ pound chicken breasts

1 cup fresh white mushrooms, sliced

½ head broccoli, cut into small florets

Directions:

Preheat the oven to 350 degrees F. Lightly, grease a baking dish.

In a bowl, mix together all ingredients except chicken, mushrooms and broccoli.

Arrange chicken in prepared baking dish and top with mushroom slices.

Place broccoli florets around chicken evenly.

Pour 1 / 2 of honey mixture over chicken and broccoli evenly.

Bake for approximately twenty minutes.

Now, coat the chicken with remaining sauce and bake for approximately 10 minutes.

Nutrition:

Calories: 427,

Fat: 9g,

Carbohydrates: 16g,

Fiber: 7g,

Protein: 35g

Phosphorus 371 mg

Potassium 501 mg

Sodium 353 mg

Gnocchi and Chicken Dumplings

Preparation Time: 10 minutes

Cooking Time: 40 minutes

Servings: 10

Ingredients:

Chicken breast – 2 pounds

Gnocchi – 1 pound

Light olive oil – ¼ cup

Better Than Bouillon® Chicken Base – 1 tablespoon

Chicken stock (reduced-sodium) – 6 cups

Fresh celery (diced finely) – ½ cup

Fresh onions (diced finely) – ½ cup

Fresh carrots (diced finely) – ½ cup

Fresh parsley (chopped) – ¼ cup

Black pepper – 1 teaspoon

Italian seasoning – 1 teaspoon

Directions:

Start by placing the stock over a high flame. Add in the oil and let it heat through.

Add the chicken to the hot oil and shallow-fry until all sides turn golden brown.

Toss in the carrots, onions, and celery and cook for about 5 minutes. Pour in the chicken stock and let it cool on a high flame for about 30 minutes.

Reduce the flame and add in the chicken bouillon, Italian seasoning, and black pepper. Stir well.

Toss in the store-bought gnocchi and let it cook for about 15 minutes. Keep stirring.

Once done, transfer into a serving bowl. Add parsley and serve hot!

Nutrition:

Protein – 28 g

Carbohydrates – 38 g

Fat – 10 g

Cholesterol – 58 mg

Sodium – 121 mg

Potassium – 485 mg

Calcium – 38 mg

Fiber – 2 g

Smoky Turkey Chili

Preparation Time: 5 minutes

Cooking Time: 45 minutes

Servings: 8

Ingredients:

12ounce lean ground turkey

1/2 red onion, chopped

2 cloves garlic, crushed and chopped

½ teaspoon of smoked paprika

½ teaspoon of chili powder

½ teaspoon of dried thyme

¼ cup reduced-sodium beef stock

½ cup of water

1 ½ cups baby spinach leaves, washed

3 wheat tortillas

Directions:

Brown the ground beef in a dry skillet over a medium-high heat.

Add in the red onion and garlic.

Sauté the onion until it goes clear.

Transfer the contents of the skillet to the slow cooker.

Add the remaining ingredients and simmer on Low for 30–45 minutes.

Stir through the spinach for the last few minutes to wilt.

Slice tortillas and gently toast under the broiler until slightly crispy.

Serve on top of the turkey chili.

Nutrition:

Calories: 93.5

Protein: 8g

Carbohydrates: 3g

Fat: 5.5g

Cholesterol: 30.5mg

Sodium: 84.5mg

Potassium: 142.5mg

Phosphorus: 92.5mg

Calcium: 29mg

Fiber: 0.5g

Conclusion

You likely had little knowledge about your kidneys before. You probably didn't know how you could take steps to improve your kidney health and decrease the risk of developing kidney failure. However, through reading this book, you now understand the power of the human kidney, as well as the prognosis of chronic kidney disease. While over thirty-million Americans are being affected by kidney disease, you can now take steps to be one of the people who is actively working to promote your kidney health.

Kidney disease now ranks as the 18th deadliest condition in the world. In the United States alone, it is reported that over 600,000 Americans succumb to kidney failure.

These stats are alarming, which is why, it is necessary to take proper care of your kidneys, starting with a kidney-friendly diet. These recipes are ideal whether you have been diagnosed with a kidney problem or you want to prevent any kidney issue.

With regards to your wellbeing and health, it's a smart thought to see your doctor as frequently as conceivable to ensure you don't run into preventable issues that you needn't get. The kidneys are your body's toxin channel (just like the liver), cleaning the blood of remote substances and toxins that are discharged from things like preservatives in food & other toxins.

At the point when you eat flippantly and fill your body with toxins, either from nourishment, drinks (liquor or alcohol for instance) or even from the air you inhale (free radicals are in the sun and move through your skin, through messy air, and numerous food sources contain them). Your body additionally will in general convert numerous things that appear to be benign until your body's organs convert them into things like formaldehyde because of a synthetic response and transforming phase.

One case of this is a large portion of those diet sugars utilized in diet soft drinks for instance, Aspartame transforms into Formaldehyde in the body. These toxins must be expelled, or they can prompt ailment, renal (kidney) failure, malignant growth, & various other painful problems.

This isn't a condition that occurs without any forethought it is a dynamic issue and in that it very well may be both found early and treated, diet changed, and settling what is causing the issue is conceivable. It's conceivable to have partial renal failure yet, as a rule; it requires some time (or downright awful diet for a short time) to arrive at absolute renal failure. You would prefer not to reach total renal failure since this will require standard dialysis treatments to save your life.

Dialysis treatments explicitly clean the blood of waste and toxins in the blood utilizing a machine in light of the fact that your body can no longer carry out the responsibility. Without treatments, you could die a very painful death. Renal failure can be the consequence of long-haul diabetes, hypertension, unreliable diet, and can stem from other health concerns.

A renal diet is tied in with directing the intake of protein and phosphorus in your eating routine. Restricting your sodium intake is likewise significant. By controlling these two variables you can control the vast majority of the toxins/waste made by your body and thus this enables your kidney to 100% function. In the event that you get this early enough and truly moderate your diets with extraordinary consideration, you could avert all-out renal failure. In the event that you get this early, you can take out the issue completely.

CPSIA information can be obtained
at www.ICGtesting.com
Printed in the USA
BVHW061340220221
600775BV00003B/14